FUNDOSCOPY IN MEDICINE

Khan & Khalid

Kindle Direct Publishing

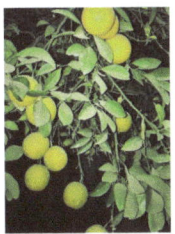

Copyright © 2023 Habibullah Khan

All rights reserved
No part of this book may be reproduced, or stored in a retrieval system, or transmitted in any form or by any means, electronic, mechanical, photocopying, recording, or otherwise, without the written permission of copyright owner.
ISBN 9798849009476
Cover design: H Khan
Published at Kindle Direct Publishing.

"And the one, who saved a life, is surely as if he had saved the whole mankind."
(Al-Quran, Sura Al-Maida; 5:32)

Dedicated to our great teachers and brilliant students.

CONTRIBUTING AUTHORS

Professor Habibullah Khan, MRCP UK, FRCP Edin
Consultant Physician, Rauf Medical Center, D.I.Khan. Former Professor of Medicine, Gomal Medical College, D.I.Khan, Pakistan

Muhammad Kamran Khalid, FCPS Ophth, FCPS VR
Associate Professor, Department of Ophthalmology, DHQ Teaching Hospital, Gomal Medical College, D.I.Khan, Pakistan

Professor Zafar Hayat, FCPS, FRCP Ire, FRCP Edin
Professor of Medicine, Kabir Medical College, Gandhara University, Peshawar, Former Professor of Medicine, Khyber Medical College, Peshawar, Pakistan

Professor Iftikhar Ahmad, PhD, DO
Consultant Ophthalmologist, Eye Clinic, and Professor of Community Medicine, Gomal Medical College, D.I.Khan, Pakistan

Nazli Gul, FCPS
Assistant Professor, Department of Ophthalmology, Hayatabad Medical Complex, Khyber Girls Medical College, Peshawar, Pakistan

Muhammad Sharjeel, FCPS
Assistant Professor, Department of Ophthalmology, MM Teaching Hospital, Gomal Medical College, D.I.Khan, Pakistan

Hafsa Habib, MBBS
Medical Officer, Provincial Health Services, KP, Pakistan

Dure Nayab, FCPS
Assistant Professor, Department of Gastroenterology & Hepatology, MM Teaching Hospital, Gomal Medical College, D.I.Khan, Pakistan

CONTENTS

Title Page
Copyright
Epigraph
Dedication
CONTRIBUTING AUTHORS
Preface
Introduction
ABBREVIATIONS

FUNDOSCOPY	1
NORMAL FUNDUS	4
VARIATIONS IN NORMAL FUNDUS	7
DIABETIC EYE DISEASE	12
HYPERTENSIVE RETINOPATHY	23
OPTIC ATROPHY	27
oPTIC NEURITIS	29
PAPILLEDEMA	30
RETINITIS PIGMENTOSA	32
TOXOPLASMOSIS	34
WILSON'S DISEASE	36
VASCULAR PATHOLOGY	39
MILIARY TUBERCULOSIS	44
INFECTIVE ENDOCARDITIS	45
HEMATOLOGICAL DISORDERS	48
SYSTEMIC LUPUS ERYTHEMATOSUS	50
CONNECTIVE TISSUE DISORDERS	52
BIBLIOGRAPHY	57
About The Author	59
Books By This Author	61

PREFACE

It is a matter of great honor and pleasure to introduce "Fundoscopy in Medicine". It may be logical to ask that in this era of internet with tremendous information available online, why was it necessary to write this book? Of course, there are dozens of scholarly-written books available on this topic but as the name of the series PEARLS OF MEDICINE" indicates, it will act as an extraordinary pearl to the already available collection.

"Fundoscopy in Medicine" is a combined effort of the physicians and ophthalmologists. Although we will mainly concentrate on the fundoscopic findings in various diseases but other ophthalmic features of these disorders and other important medical aspects will also be briefly touched.

This short book will be of interest to the medical students, postgraduate trainees and clinicians alike and hopefully, this effort will be appreciated by both the "internal medicine" and "ophthalmic" community.

Research and publication are the ongoing processes which enhance our knowledge. A tiny effort of today may become the brilliant history for tomorrow and we should struggle in this world of survival of the fittest and the kindest to share our knowledge and experience with our colleagues.

The book is mainly illustrative with just a brief account in the form of text. The purpose is to keep the interest of our busy readers and act like a mnemonic for those who are going soon to appear in their final exams. It will both be available as print and e-book.

We have incorporated important references to the most recent quality reviews and original research articles in the bibliography. The popular books and databases on this topic were of course thoroughly consulted while writing.

We are grateful to all our colleagues for their support and encouragement. This edition would not have been possible without their help. Last but not the least, special thanks to our patient families for their constant support.

We hope "Fundoscopy in Medicine" will prove to be the best friend of clinicians and students not only in the Internal Medicine but in the Ophthalmology as well.

Suggestions from our precious readers would be highly appreciated and honored for improvements in the future editions.

The Editor
Habibullah Khan, FRCP Edin
E-mail: pearlsofmedicine@gmail.com
Twitter: @Medicinepearls

INTRODUCTION

The value of fundoscopy in Medicine is well-established and every physician is expected to use an ophthalmoscope properly. As a matter of fact many systemic diseases present with typical changes in the eyes especially the fundi. Identification of these changes may not only help in the diagnosis but also the subsequent follow-up of these patients.

In this book the diseases having fundoscopic and other associated ophthalmic manifestations are briefly discussed with colored illustrations.

ABBREVIATIONS

ACR	American College of Rheumatology
BIH	Benign intracranial hypertension
BRAO	Branch retinal artery occlusion
BP	Blood pressure
CCB	Calcium channel blocker
CNS	Central nervous system
CT	Computerized tomography
DKA	Diabetic ketoacidosis
DM	Diabetes mellitus
DR	Diabetic retinopathy
EDS	Ehlers Danlos syndrome
FBS	Fasting blood sugar
FFA	Fundus fluorescein angiogram
HIV	Human immunodeficiency virus
HT	Hypertension
IE	Infective endocarditis
JNC	Joint National Committee on prevention, detection, evaluation and treatment of high blood pressure
KF ring	Kayser Fleischer ring
MRI	Magnetic resonance imaging
MS	Multiple sclerosis
MVP	Mitral valve prolapse
OA	Optic atrophy
PDR	Proliferative diabetic retinopathy
RBS	Random blood sugar
RP	Retinitis pigmentosa
SBE	Subacute bacterial endocarditis
SLE	Systemic lupus erythematosus
SOL	Space occupying lesion
TB	Tuberculosis

FUNDOSCOPY

Khalid K

Examination of the ocular fundus or fundoscopy is an integral part of ophthalmic examination and its importance in the Internal Medicine can't be underestimated. Many systemic diseases present with characteristic changes in the ocular fundus. These changes may help in the diagnosis and follow-up of various disorders.

The value of fundoscopy in Medicine is so well-established that every physician is expected to be able to use an ophthalmoscope properly. Fundoscopy is considered by many as part and parcel of the general physical examination.

In the forthcoming sections of this book the diseases having fundoscopic and other associated ophthalmic manifestations are briefly discussed with more emphasis on the colored illustrations especially of the fundus.

OPHTHALMOSCOPE

Ophthalmoscope is an instrument to examine the ocular fundi. It's proper use is an art that can only be acquired by practice. (Fig. 1)

Ophthalmoscopy or fundoscopy means to examine the ocular fundus. It can be direct or indirect.

In internal medicine, direct ophthalmoscopy is usually used. It provides a magnified view of the ocular fundus.

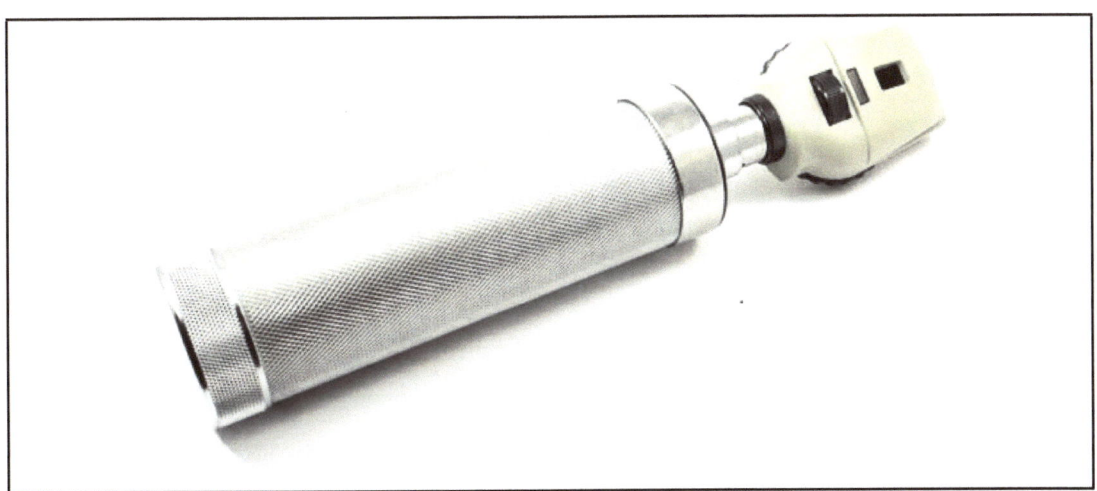

Figure 1: Standard size ophthalmoscope.

Ophthalmoscope is portable and ophthalmoscopy can easily be performed at the bedside by a general physician.

The technique of proper fundoscopy can be learnt with little effort. Time should be given for dilatation of the pupils to get maximum information. Mydriatic eye drops like tropicamide is used for this purpose. One drop 2-3 times at 5-7 minutes interval is instilled to dilate the pupils enough to examine the posterior pole.

Hold the scope in your right hand for the right and left hand for the left eye. Also use the respective eye for the purpose.

Switch on and adjust the suitable resolution depending upon your refractive error and thus the number of your glasses. (Fig. 2)

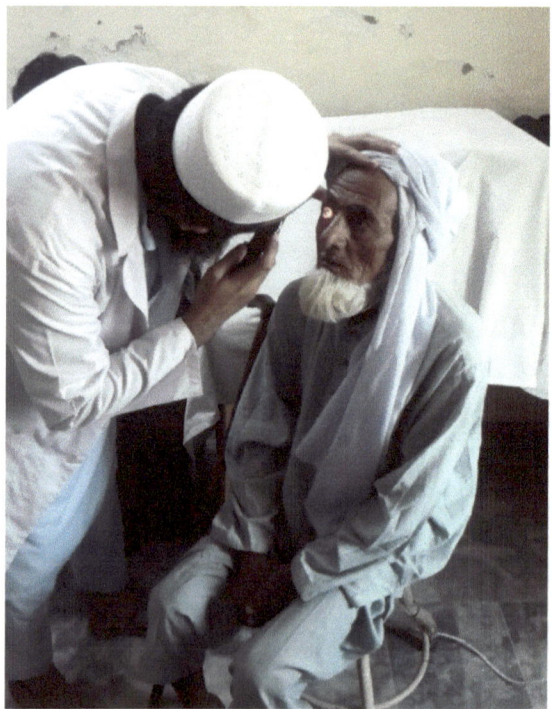

Figure 2: Direct ophthalmoscopy in progress.
(Photograph by Khalid K)

Before starting examination, instructions should be given to the patient to look straight ahead and not to move his/her eyes as the examiner's head blocks the view.

Locate the optic nerve head by following the course of major retinal vessels. Temporal to the optic nerve head lies the macula.

Most of the important fundus structures are lying at the posterior pole i.e. optic nerve head, macula and major retinal vessels and can be easily examined in a short time.

For more detailed and peripheral fundus examination the patient should be referred to an ophthalmologist if required.

NORMAL FUNDUS

Ahmad I

Fundus is the internal surface of the eye and includes the following structures:

- Retina
- Optic disc
- Macula
- Fovea
- Posterior pole

Retina is the only part of central nervous system (CNS) visible from outside. Like-wise, the fundus is the only site where vasculature can be directly visualized and assessed.

Viewing the fundus is a way to get information regarding the patient's overall vascular status and certain pathological processes otherwise invisible e.g. diabetes, hypertension, and raised intra cranial pressure.

The fundus can be examined by an ophthalmoscope &/or a fundus camera.

Dilated fundus examination makes the use of short-acting mydriatic eye drops to dilate the pupil to obtain a better view as compared to non-dilated examination. (Fig. 3 a & b)

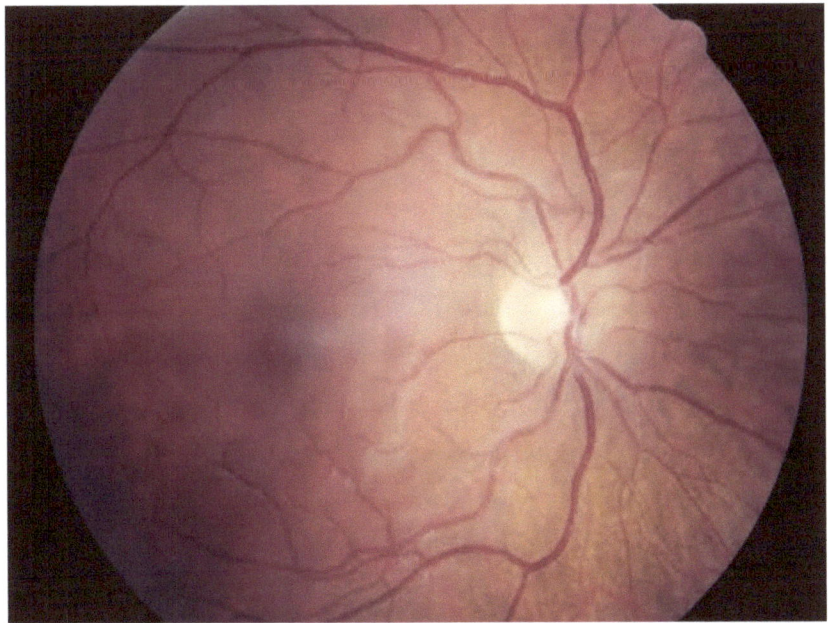

Figure 3(a): Normal fundus showing the optic disc, macula, and retinal vessels.
(Photograph by Sharjeel M)

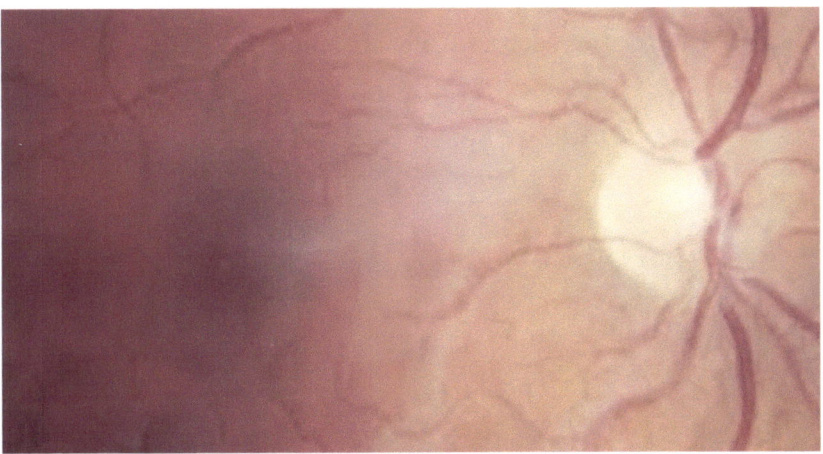

Figure 3(b): Normal fundus - closer view of the optic disc and macula.
(Photograph by Sharjeel M)

The color of the fundus is red. The macula is in the center and the optic disc is located towards the nose.

The optic disc is like a doughnut with a pink neuroretinal rim and a central white depression, the physiologic cup. Neuroretinal rim transmits the axons of the retinal ganglion cells. It turns white in inflammation, infarction, and compression due to death of axons. The distinct margins of the optic disc may be blurred in papilledema and the rim rises well above the retinal surface. Common causes of disc edema are increased intracranial pressure, optic neuritis and infarction. The horizontal diameter of the physiological cup should not exceed half the horizontal diameter of the entire disc (cup-to-disc ratio). Otherwise, suspect pathologic optic disc cupping is suspected as in glaucoma. The retinal arteries and veins come out from the optic disc. Vessels directed nasally have a radial course, while those directed temporally have an arching course.

The arteries are brighter red and narrower than veins. The retinal arteries lack a muscular coat and are more rightly called arterioles.

The macula is located about two disc-diameters temporal to the optic disc. It looks slightly darker than the surrounding retina because of increased pigment. The fovea, a 2.5 mm diameter area, lies in the center of the macular region. It is made-up exclusively of cones, and possesses the high-contrast discriminative vision and color vision.

VARIATIONS IN NORMAL FUNDUS

Sharjeel M

There are lots of variations normally seen in the fundus which should not be confused with pathology. The less experienced ones specially the medical residents may confuse it with the disease.

Some of the commonly encountered variations are given below:

- Myelinated nerve fibers

- Tigroid retina

- Retinal nevus

- Tilted disc

MYELINATED NERVE FIBERS

Nerve fibres in the retina are normally unmyelinated and transparent. Sometimes myelinated nerve fibers from the optic nerve extend as whitish feather-like lesions radiating from the optic disc. This is a harmless finding and doesn't signify a disease. (Fig. 4)

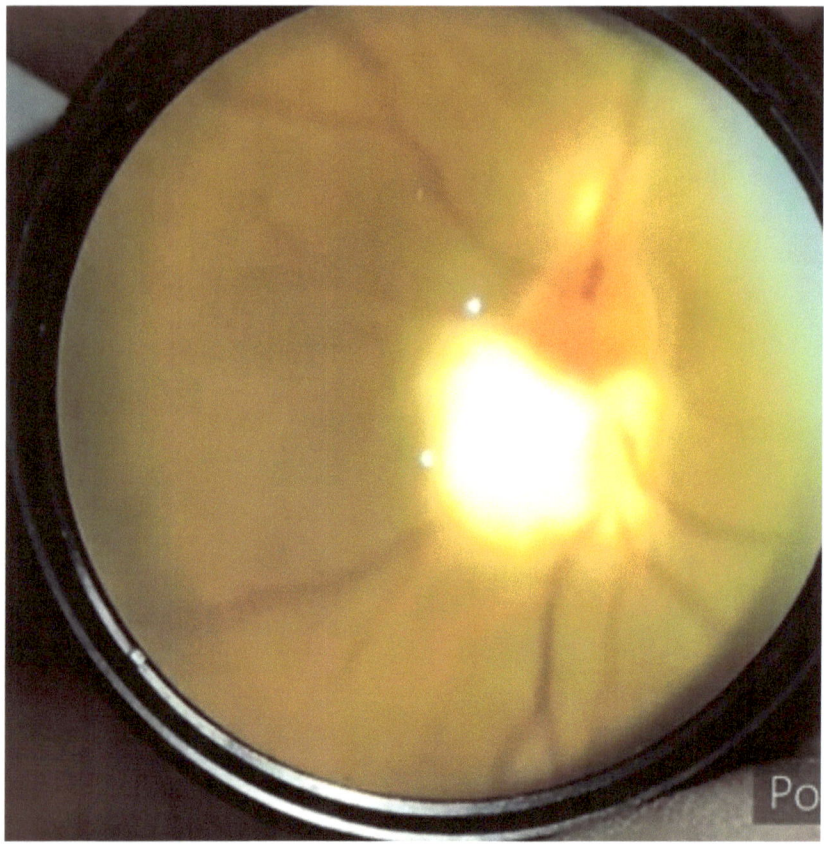

Figure 4: Myelinated nerve fibers radiating from the optic disc.
(Fundus photograph by Sharjeel M)

TIGROID RETINA

In high myopia the fundus may look abnormal. The retina is thinned due to stretching of the sclera which may present as "tigroid retina". (Fig. 5) High myopia may rarely lead to choroidal neovascularization which may result in retinal detachment.

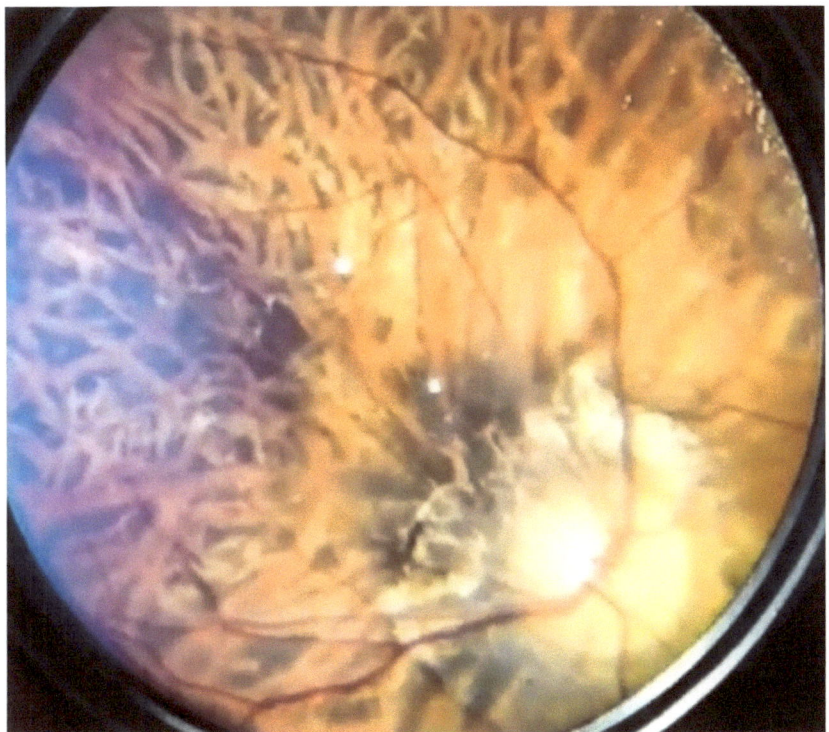

Figure 5: Tigroid retina.
(Fundus photograph by Sharjeel M)

RETINAL NEVUS

Nevi as normally seen on the skin can sometimes also be seen in the fundus. (Fig. 6) This is a harmless finding that just needs follow-up for any rapid growth to rule out melanoma.

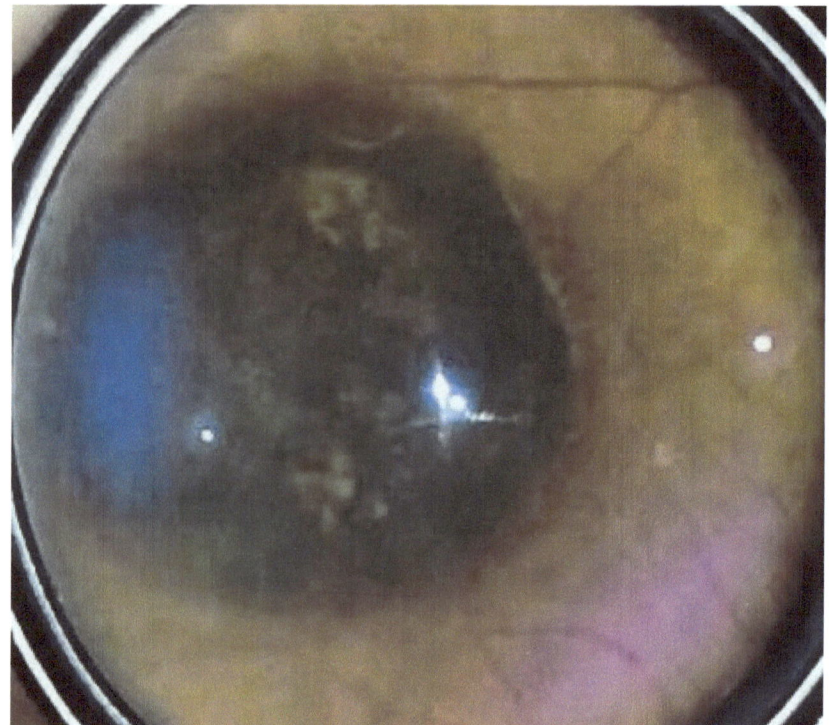

Figure 6: Close-up view of a retinal nevus.
(Fundus photograph by Imtiaz HS)

TILTED DISC

Optic disc is normally round or oval but sometimes the disc may look tilted. (Fig. 7) Tilted disc can be an isolated normal variation or it may be associated with the spectrum of high myopia.

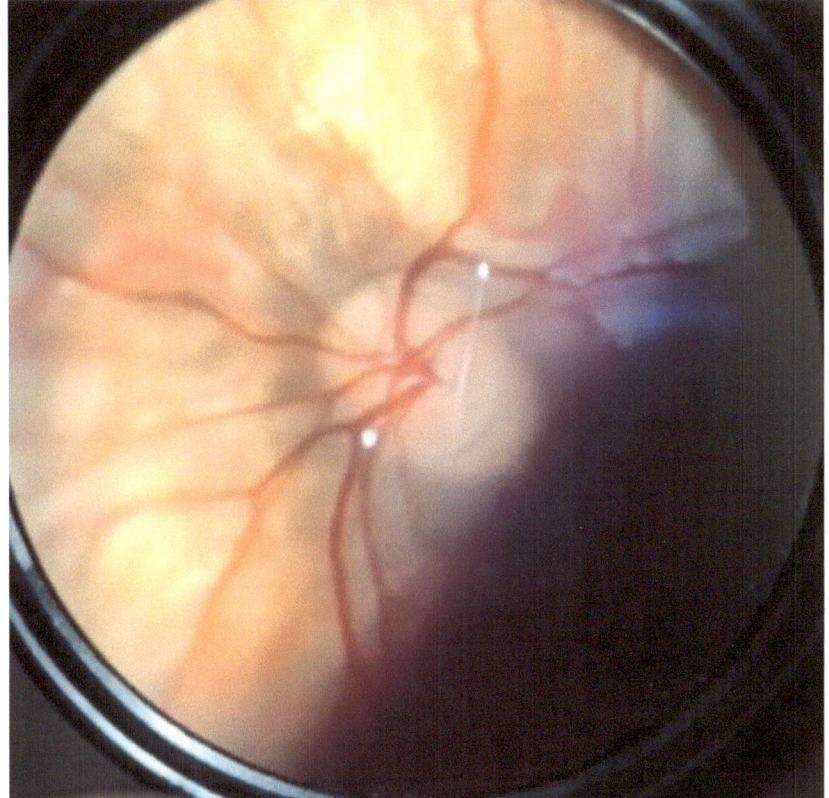

Figure 7: Fundus of a patient with tilted disc.
(Photograph by Sharjeel M)

DIABETIC EYE DISEASE

Khan H

Diabetes mellitus (DM) is a metabolic disorder caused by deficiency or inefficiency of insulin, resulting in abnormal carbohydrates, lipids and proteins metabolism, characterized by hyperglycemia.

Generally, it is classified as type 1 and type 2. Polyuria, polydipsia, and weight-loss are its classical presenting features. It is important to note that type 1 diabetes may present for the first time with its most serious complication, diabetic ketoacidosis (DKA) in upto 25% of cases.

DM is notorious for its complications which could be acute or chronic.

Acute complications include DKA, hypoglycemia, hyperosmolar state and lactic acidosis.

Chronic complications are mainly vascular, both micro and macrovascular.

Microvascular complications include retinopathy, neuropathy, and nephropathy.

Macrovascular complications are cerebrovascular, coronary, and peripheral vascular disease.

Increased susceptibility to infections, especially of the urinary tract, skin and respiratory tract is also a problem.

Diabetic foot is a serious complication and involves multiple factors, including vasculopathy, neuropathy, mechanical factors and defective immune status.

Skin lesions due to diabetes apart from infections include diabetic dermopathy, and necrobiosis lipoidica diabeticorum.

Diabetes can affect the eyes in various ways. It can cause retinopathy and can lead to early cataracts. (Fig. 8) Due to increased susceptibility to infections panophthalmitis is more common in these patients as compared to the normal population.

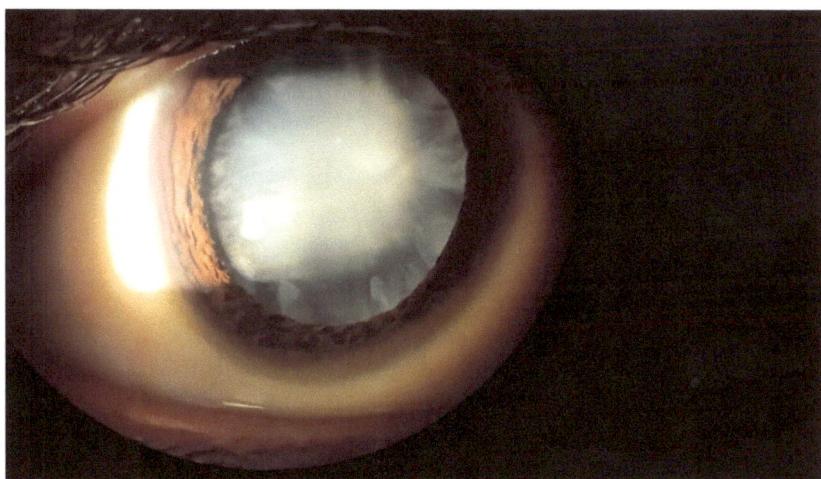

Figure 8: Slit lamp examination in a 40 years old diabetic showing an early mature cataract.
(Photograph by Sharjeel M)

DIABETIC RETINOPATHY

Retinopathy is a serious complication of diabetes. It is a chronic, progressive and potentially sight-threatening condition of the retinal microvasculature.

Its prevalence and severity depends upon various factors. The risk factors for progression of diabetic retinopathy are given below. (Table 1)

The main threat to vision in diabetic retinopathy comes from:

1. Neovascularization leading to intraocular hemorrhage, fibrosis, and possible retinal detachment.

2. Damage to the macula /fovea with loss of central visual acuity.

FACTORS PREDISPOSING OR AGGRAVATING DIABETIC RETINOPATHY

	Factors	Remarks
1	Poor glycemic control	Poor glycemic control predisposes, while good control can delay the onset and slow the progression of diabetic retinopathy.
2	Hypertension	Effective BP control reduces the risk of retinopathy progression and visual acuity deterioration.
3	Duration of diabetes	Risk of developing diabetic retinopathy or its progression increases over time. After 15 years, 80% of Type 1 diabetics will have retinopathy. After 19 years, up to 84% patients with type 2 diabetes will have retinopathy.
4	Dyslipidemia	Elevated blood lipid levels can lead to greater accumulation of exudates. This condition is associated with a higher risk of moderate visual loss.
5	Ethnicity	Certain ethnic groups are more likely to have diabetes. These include African Americans, Latinos and Native Americans.
6	Pregnancy	Risk and progression of diabetic retinopathy increases in pregnancy. However, some studies have suggested that with treatment these changes are reversed after delivery and there is no increase in long-term progression of disease.

Table 1: Factors predisposing or aggravating diabetic retinopathy.

CLASSIFICATION

Diabetic retinopathy is classified according to the fundoscopic findings. Historically, it is based on the signs of increasing severity, ranking from no retinopathy through various stages of background, preproliferative, proliferative, and advanced proliferative disease. However, this grading may not accurately reflect the functional severity of disease since maculopathy with severe visual loss can occur with only background changes at the macula. As a consequence, two different approaches to classification have emerged:

1. Those designed to cover the full range of retinopathy aimed for ophthalmologists.
2. Those for screening, aimed mainly for internists.

The simple classification of diabetic retinopathy on the basis of the presence or absence of neovascularisation is practical for screening. (Table 2)

DIABETIC RETINOPATHY

Grading	Changes
Non-proliferative	Microaneurysms Hard exudates
Pre-proliferative	Retinal hemorrhages Soft exudates
Proliferative	Neovascularisation Fibrosis Complications

Table 2: Classification of diabetic retinopathy.

BACKGROUND RETINOPATHY

In background diabetic retinopathy, there are hard exudates and dot hemorrhages. Hard exudates are actually lipid deposits and dot hemorrhages are microaneurysms. (Fig. 9)

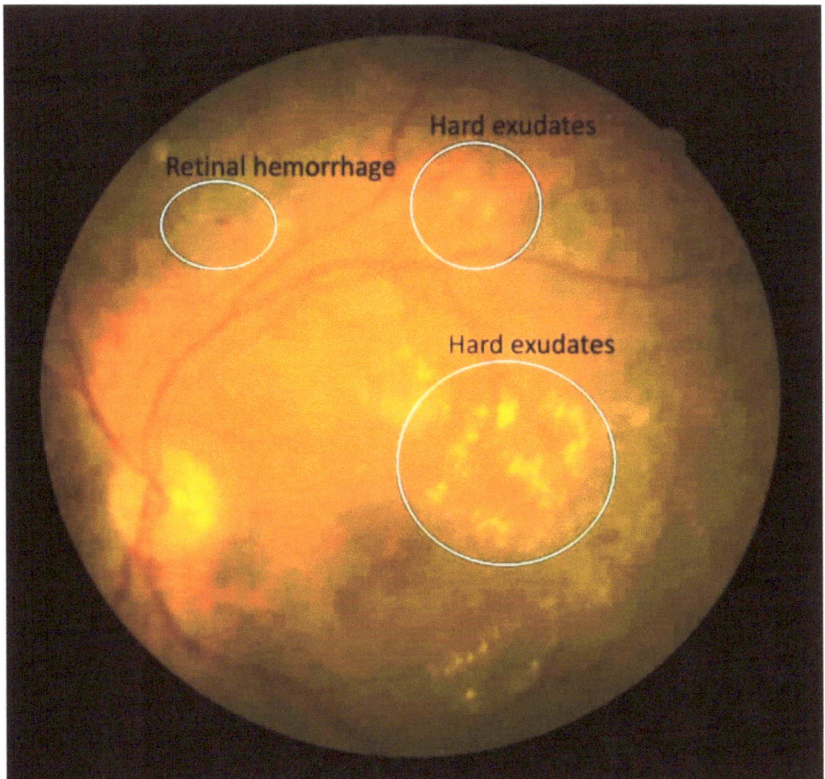

Figure 9: Background diabetic retinopathy with dot hemorrhages and hard exudates. Hard exudates are seen at the macula (maculopathy) and elsewhere.
(Fundus photograph by Gul N)

PRE-PROLIFERATIVE RETINOPATHY

This is the stage where although proliferative changes i.e. neovascularization which is a threat for vision have not yet occurred but there is ischemia of retina which predisposes the patient to proliferative changes. There are soft exudates and hemorrhages along with the background changes. (Fig. 10)

Laser therapy at this stage may prevent its progression to proliferative stage.

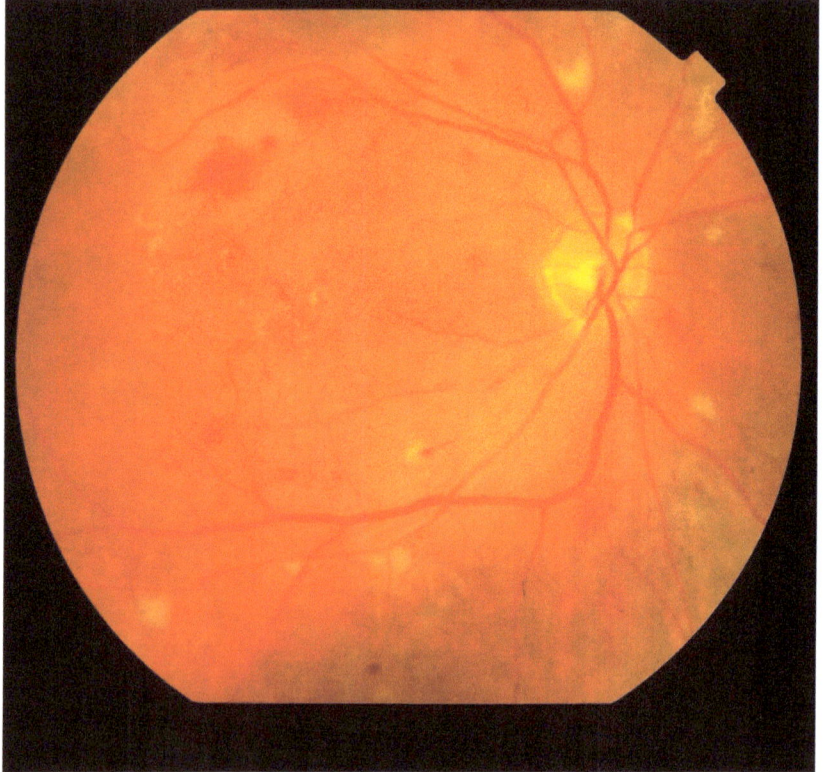

Figure 10: Pre-proliferative diabetic retinopathy showing soft exudates and hemorrhages along with background changes.
(Fundus photograph by Khalid K)

PROLIFERATIVE RETINOPATHY

Neovascularization is the hallmark of proliferative diabetic retinopathy (PDR) which is a consequence of retinal ischemia. These new vessels are fragile and may lead to serious hemorrhages and fibrosis in the vitreous which may further predispose the eye to more serious complications like retinal detachment. (Fig. 11, 12)

Duration of diabetes is a strong predictor for the development of proliferative diabetic retinopathy.

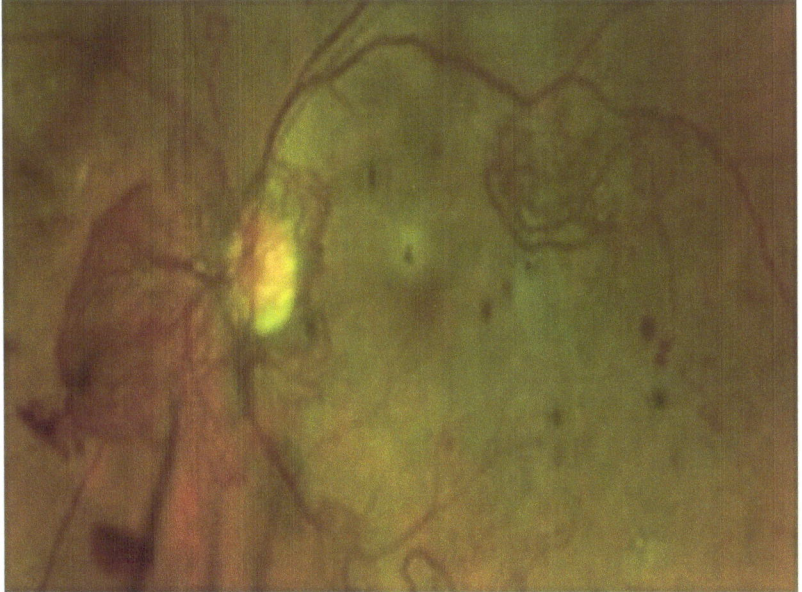

Figure 11 (a): Advanced proliferative diabetic retinopathy with neovascularization and fibrosis at the disc and elsewhere.

(Fundus photograph by Gul N)

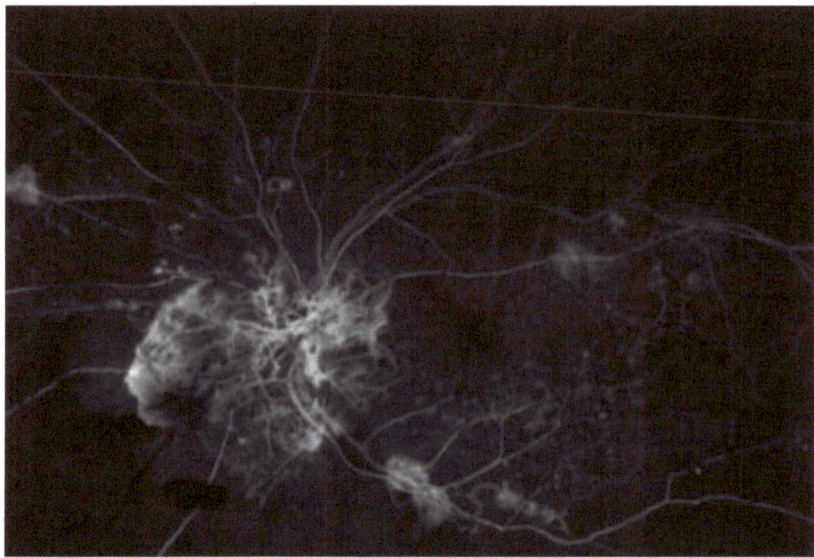

Figure 11 (b): Corresponding Fundus Fluorescein Angiogram (FFA) showing leakage from the new vessels as evidenced by hyperfluorescence at the disc and elsewhere. There is also extensive retinal ischemia as shown by the capillary drop outs.
(Fundus photograph by Gul N)

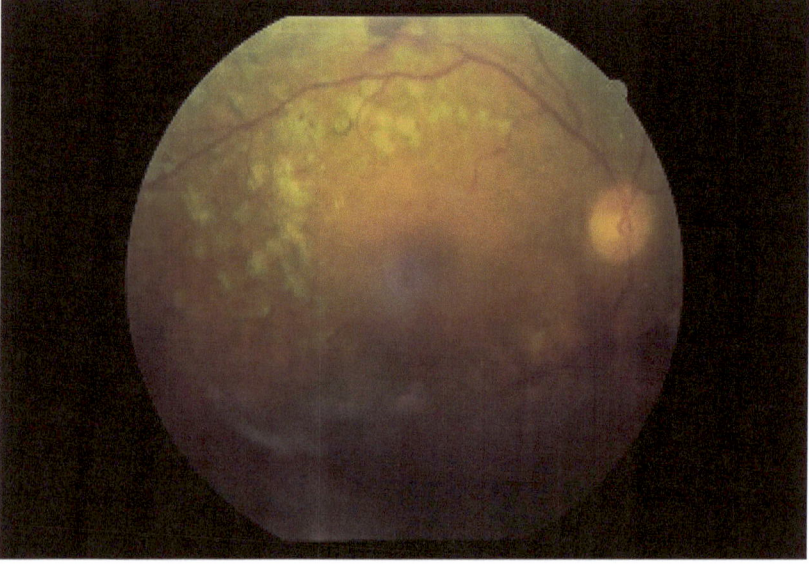

Figure 12: Laser mark at the periphery of the fundus in a patient with diabetic retinopathy.
(Fundus photograph by Khalid K)

MACULOPATHY

Macula or its center, the fovea is the center of vision and any pathology at this area may be detrimental for the vision. That is why even the non-proliferative changes in this area are taken as seriously as proliferative changes in the rest of the retina. (Fig. 13)

Diabetic maculopathy is the most common cause of visual impairment in diabetic patients. It can be focal, diffuse or mixed.

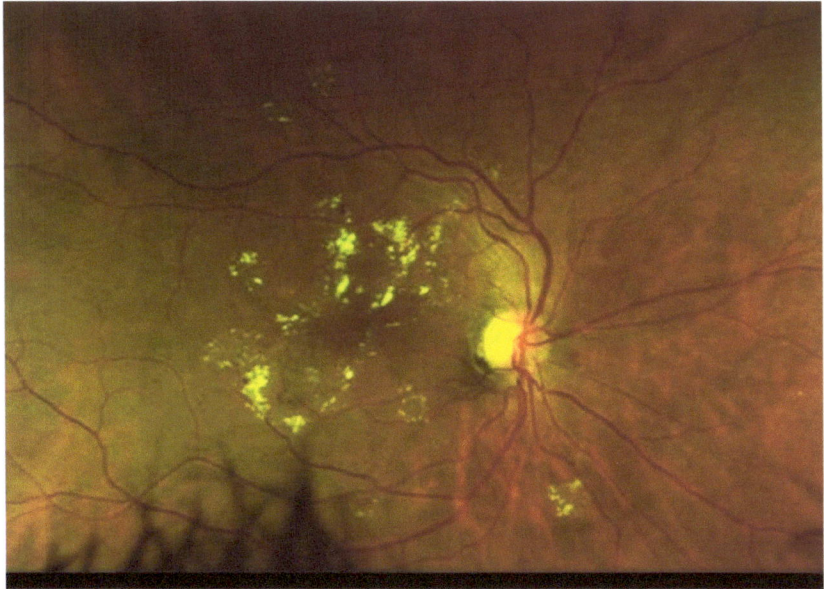

Figure 13: Diabetic maculopathy showing rings of hard exudates at the macula.
(Fundus photograph by Gul N)

MANAGEMENT

Tight glycaemic control:

Contol of blood sugar levels (FBS <130 mg/dl, RBS <160 mg/dl, HbA1C <7%) has a pivotal role in the management of DM.

It can be achieved by life style changes (Diet & Exercise) and hypoglycemic agents (Insulin &/or oral antidiabetics).

Photocoagulation:

Laser therapy is the most effective treatment for preproliferative, and proliferative changes.

It prevents the complications by preventing the neovascularization.

It is also advisable for patients with maculopathy. Even the background changes when they involve the macula require photocoagulation.

BP control, Lipid correction, & antiplatelet therapy:

In certain cases where required.

Intravitreal anti-VEGF:

Injections of anti Vascular Endothelial Growth Factor (VEGF) are advisable for macular edema.

Surgical intervention:

Viterectomy may be required in certain cases.

Cataract extraction is performed when needed.

HYPERTENSIVE RETINOPATHY

Hayat Z

Hypertension (HT) is defined as persistent elevation of blood pressure (BP) to a level at which pharmacological management will benefit the patient.

According to the 8th report of the Joint National Committee for Prevention, Detection & Treatment of Hypertension (JNC-8), this level is $\geq$140/90 mmHg for adults below 60 and $\geq$150/90 mmHg for $\geq$60 years age.

For persons with chronic kidney disease (CKD) or diabetes, there is no difference in the diagnostic BP and target BP for control.

HT can lead to myocardial infarction, stroke, renal failure, and death if not detected and treated well in time.

Fundoscopy is helpful to check the effects of HT on the vasculature.

Normally, the retinal arteries are brighter red and narrower than veins. In hypertensive retinopathy arteriolar constriction is seen as "silver wiring" and tortuosity.

Hypertensive retinopathy is graded on the basis of "*Keith, Wagener, & Barker* classification". (Table 3) Changes of hypertensive retinopathy are shown in the Fig. 14.

KEITH, WAGENER & BARKER CLASSIFICATION

Grade	Features
I	Slight or modest narrowing of retinal arterioles, AV ratio ≥ 1:2.
II	Modest to severe narrowing of retinal arterioles, AV ratio < 1:2 or AV nicking.
III	Soft exudates and flame-shaped hemorrhages.
IV	Grade III changes + bilateral papilledema.

Table 3: Keith, Wagener & Barker classification of hypertensive retinopathy.

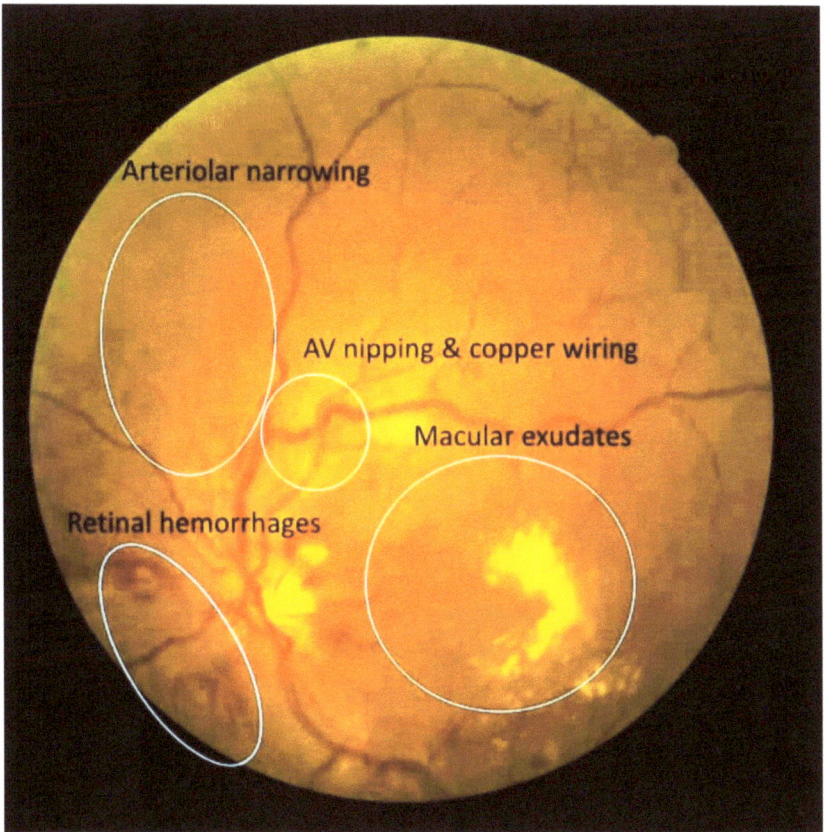

Figure 14: Grade 3 hypertensive retinopathy showing arteriolar narrowing and soft exudates.
(Fundus photograph by Gul N)

MANAGEMENT

Non-pharmacologic:

Non-pharmacological measures are not less important than the pharmacological treatment. These include:

- Dietary restrictions
- Regular exercise
- Cessation of smoking
- Optimisation of alcohol
- Weight control

Pharmacologic:

tHE Key points for practice according to the JNC-8 are given below:

- In the general population, pharmacologic treatment should be initiated when BP is ≥150/90 mmHg in adults ≥60 years, or ≥140/90 mmHg in younger than 60.

- In patients with HT and DM, pharmacologic treatment should be initiated when BP is ≥140/90 mm Hg, regardless of age.

- Initial antihypertensive treatment should include a thiazide diuretic, CCB, ACE inhibitor, or ARB in the general nonblack population or a thiazide diuretic or CCB in the general black population.

- If the target BP is not reached within one month after initiating therapy, the dosage of initial medication should be increased, or a second one added.

OPTIC ATROPHY

Ahmad I

Optic atrophy (OA) is the final common morphologic endpoint of any disease process that causes axonal degeneration in the retino-geniculate pathway.

CAUSES

There are many causes of optic atrophy; the common ones are listed below:

Congenital:
- Leber's hereditary optic neuropathy
- Autosomal dominant optic atrophy

Damage within the eye:
- Glaucoma
- Papilledema
- Optic neuritis: e.g. MS, Neuromyelitis optica

Damage along the optic nerve:
- Anterior cranial fossa tumor
- Neurodegenerative disorders
- Trauma

CLINICAL FEATURES

Symptoms include blurring of vision and defective color vision, and peripheral vision.

Fundoscopy reveals pallor of the optic disc with sharp margins, and cupping. (Fig. 6.1)

TREATMENT

Depends upon the underlying cause.

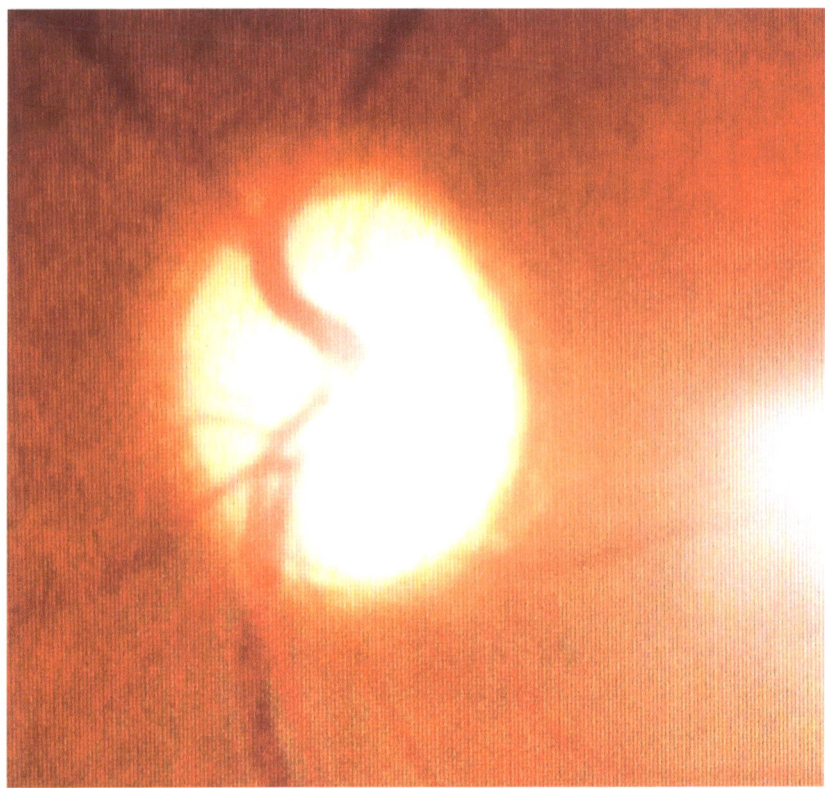

Figure 15: Optic atrophy as evident by pallor of the optic disc with sharp margins and cupping.
(Fundus photograph by Sharjeel M)

OPTIC NEURITIS

Ahmad I

Inflammation of the optic nerve or optic neuritis can occur in a variety of conditions. Symptoms include subacute visual loss and painful eye movement in one eye, with weaker direct pupillary light reflex on that side.
Fundoscopy reveals blurring of the disc margins. (Fig. 16)
Optic neuritis can be seen in conditions like multiple sclerosis (MS).

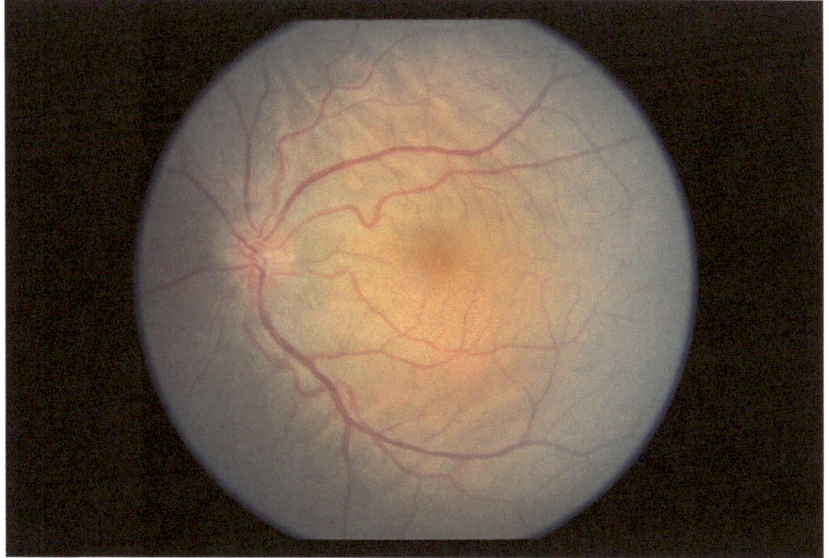

Figure 16: Optic neuritis with blurring of the margins of optic disc.
(Fundus photograph by Khalid K)

PAPILLEDEMA

Ahmad I

Raised intracranial pressure due to any reason results to papilledema. In this condition the disc margins are blurred and there is hyperemia. (Fig. 17)

Optic neuritis with blurred disc margins can be confused with papilledema. However, contrary to optic neuritis papilledema is almost always bilateral except in the rare case of anterior cranial fossa tumor which may cause optic atrophy on the ipsilateral side due to optic nerve compression and papilledema on contralateral side due to raised intracranial pressure – Foster Kenedy syndrome.

Also there is no hyperemia of the fundus in retinitis.

CAUSES

The most serious cause of papilledema is any space occupying lesion (SOL) of the head resulting in raised intracranial pressure.

Other causes include benign intracranial hypertension (BIH) which commonly occurs in young, obese ladies.

CLINICAL FEATURES

Papilledema, developing within days or weeks, initially may present without visual symptoms. Blurring of the vision, diplopia, or complete visual loss are the symptoms, depending upon the cause.

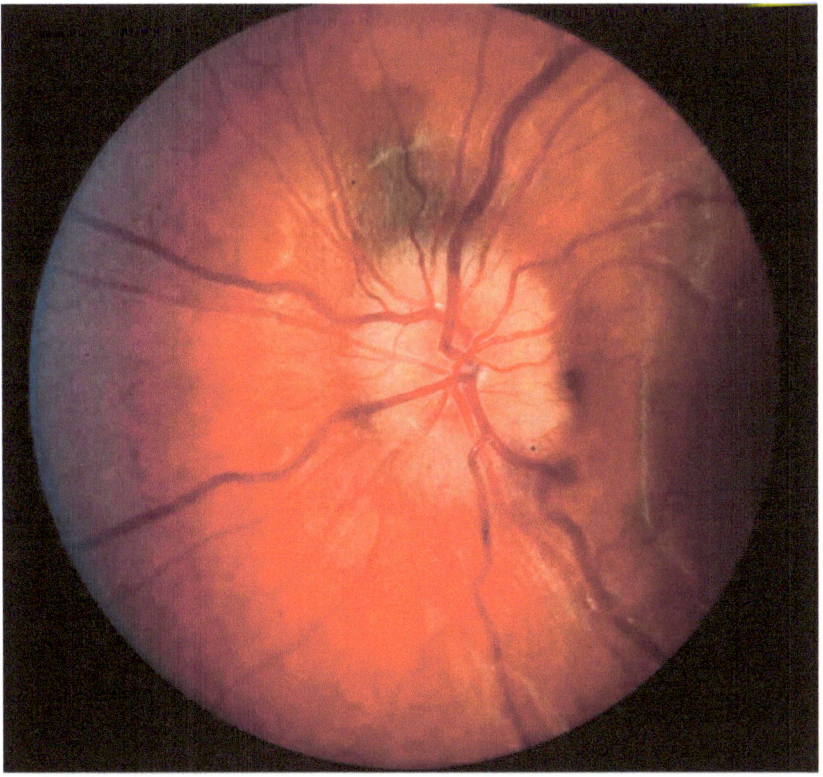

Figure 17: Papilledema: the margins of optic disc are blurred and there is hyperemia.
(Fundus photograph by Gul N)

RETINITIS PIGMENTOSA

Khan H

Retinitis pigmentosa (RP) is an autosomal recessive hereditary disorder of the retina. It is the most common inherited disease of the retina with a prevalence of 1 in 3500 to 4500 persons. Because of its easy availability, RP is shown quite often in the clinical exams.

Its characteristic features are night blindness and visual loss initially peripheral which may later become central.

Detailed family history and examination of the family members is mandatory. Drug history is important to rule out the toxicity of certain medications.

On fundoscopy, there are bony spicule-like pigmentary lesions, mostly in the periphery of the retina. (Fig. 18)

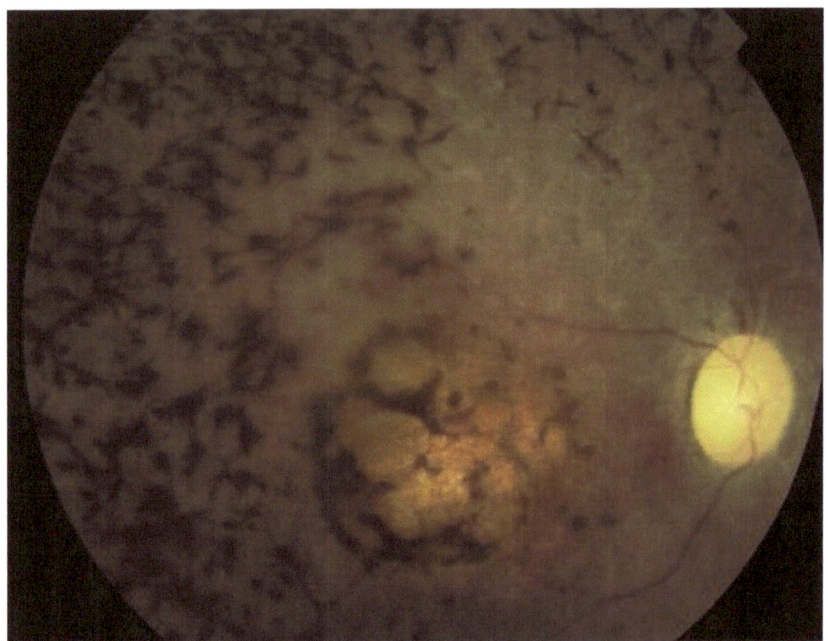

Figure 18: Typical bony spicule-like pigmentary lesions in the periphery of retina in a patient with retinitis pigmentosa.
(Fundus photograph by Khalid K)

Systemic examination may reveal syndromes with pigmentary retinopathy as a feature, such as:

- Syndromes with RP and hearing loss: Usher syndrome, Waardenburg syndrome, Alport syndrome, Refsum disease.
- Kearns-Sayre syndrome: External ophthalmoplegia, lid ptosis, heart block, and pigmentary retinopathy.
- Abetalipoproteinemia: Fat malabsorption, fat-soluble vitamin deficiencies, spinocerebellar degeneration, and pigmentary retinopathy.
- Mucopolysaccharidoses (e.g. Hurler syndrome, Scheie syndrome, Sanfilippo syndrome): Can also have pigmentary retinopathy.
- Bardet-Biedl syndrome: Polydactyly, truncal obesity, kidney dysfunction, short stature, and pigmentary retinopathy.
- Neuronal ceroid lipofuscinosis: Dementia, seizures, and pigmentary retinopathy; infantile form is known as Jansky-Bielschowsky disease, juvenile form Vogt-Spielmeyer-Batten disease, and adult form Kufs syndrome.

There is no cure for RP but patients can be helped by maximizing the available vision with refraction and low-vision evaluation.

Surgical management generally involves cataract extraction.

Retinal implant can be considered in adults with severe RP.

Drugs used include vitamin A, E, C, calcium-channel blockers, and carbonic anhydrase inhibitors.

Drugs with pigmentary retinitis as a potential adverse effect are to be avoided; like isotretinoin, sildenafil, phenothiazine, and high-dose vitamin E.

TOXOPLASMOSIS

Khan H

Toxoplasmosis is a parasitic disease caused by *Toxoplasma gondii*. It can be congenital or acquired. It is basically a systemic infestation affecting the eyes as well. Acquired disease typically occurs due to ingestion of undercooked meat contaminated with cysts of *T. gondii*. Water contaminated with oocysts is also an important source of infestation.

In the eyes, it causes necrotizing retinochoroiditis which may lead to the formation of thick vitreous strands and membranes.

Macular edema may also be seen. Elevated intraocular pressure reflects the severity of inflammation.

As the lesion heals, it appears as punched-out scar, revealing the underlying white sclera with variable pigment proliferation. (Fig. 19)

MANAGEMENT

Triple therapy with Pyrimethamine + Sulfadiazine + Prednisone for 4-6 weeks with folinic acid to avoid hematologic complications of pyrimethamine.

Quadruple therapy: Triple therapy + Clindamycin.

For prophylaxis of recurrence: Cotrimoxazole every 3 days.

During pregnancy, Spiramycin can be used in the first and early second trimester, while triple therapy later on.

Topical corticosteroids are used depending upon the anterior chamber reaction.

Depot steroids are contraindicated as it may compromise the immune response, leading to extensive necrosis and potential blindness. However, systemic corticosteroids are used to minimize the collateral damage from inflammation.

Topical cycloplegic agents can be used depending upon the anterior chamber reaction and degree of pain.

Intravitreal clindamycin and dexamethasone is used as salvage therapy in those not responding to oral treatment.

Photocoagulation, cryotherapy, and vitrectomy can be employed by vitreoretinal specialist in selected cases.

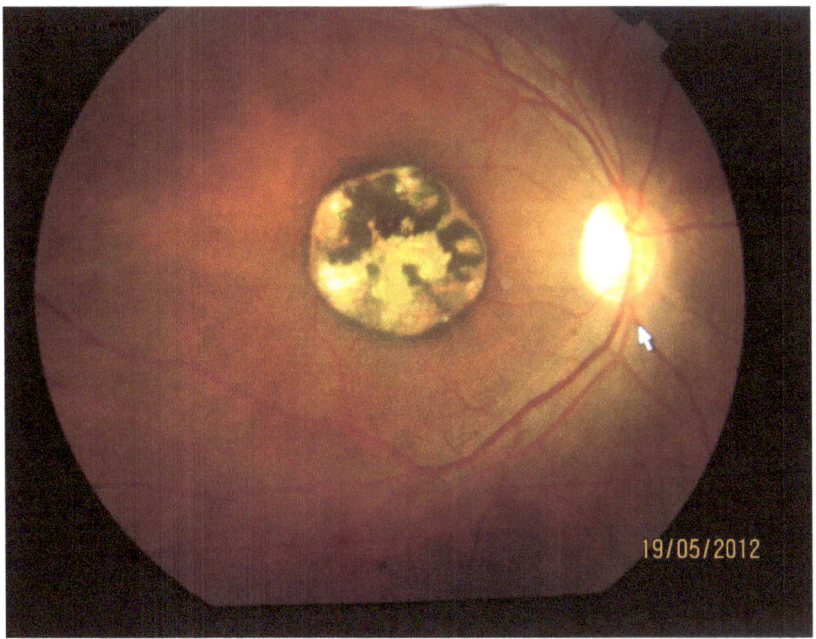

Figure 19: Optic fundus showing scar of choroido-retinitis due to toxoplasmosis.
(Picture by Khalid K)

WILSON'S DISEASE

Nayab D

Wilson's disease is an autosomal recessive disorder of copper metabolism, resulting in deposition of copper in the cornea, brain, and liver.

Its incidence is 1 in 40,000 and prevalence 29/million/year. Patients usually present at the age of 5 to 35 years.

The commonest presentation is with CNS effects like rigidity, tremor, chorea, dysarthria, seizures, and mental deterioration.

Acute hepatitis and cirrhosis may also develop.

DIAGNOSIS

The diagnosis is based on the clinical suspicion and demonstration of copper in the tissues like cornea (KF ring) or liver (biopsy with copper content).

Plasma ceruloplasmin level is low and serum copper & 24 hours urinary copper may be high.

MANAGEMENT

Chelating agents:

Penicillamine is given to reduce the copper load with pyridoxine supplement to avoid vitamin B6 deficiency.

Trientine is the second-line drug for those who can't tolerate penicillamine. It is less toxic with similar efficacy.

Dietary restrictions:

Avoid liver, mushrooms, chocolates, nuts, legumes, and shellfish.

Check the copper content of any nutritional supplement and drinking water.

Zinc sulphate supplements:

It reduces the intestinal copper transport. It is best used in asymptomatic patients. However it can be used in conjunction with chelation therapy but given 4–5 hours apart from chelators.

PROGNOSIS

Early diagnosis and effective treatment improves the outlook.

Neurological damages are mostly irreversible.

Fulminant hepatic failure may need liver transplant.

KAYSER FLEISCHER RING

Kayser Fleischer (KF) ring is a brown pigmentation in the periphery of cornea due to copper deposition. It is usually suspected visually and confirmed by slit-lamp examination. (Fig. 20 a & b)

KF ring is present in 90% patients with neurological and <50% with hepatic disease.

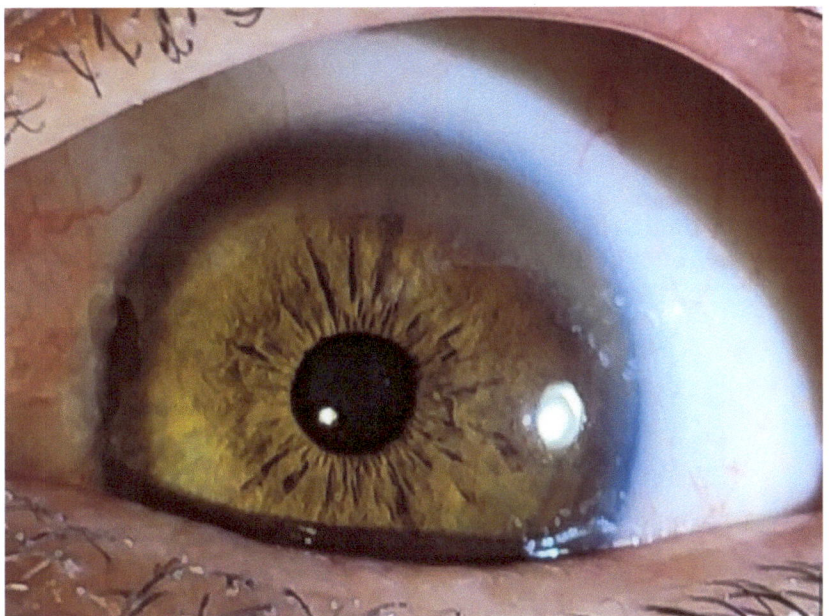

Figure 20 (a): Kayser Fleischer ring visible as a brown ring at the corneoscleral junction in a patient with Wilson's disease.

(Photograph by Sharjeel)

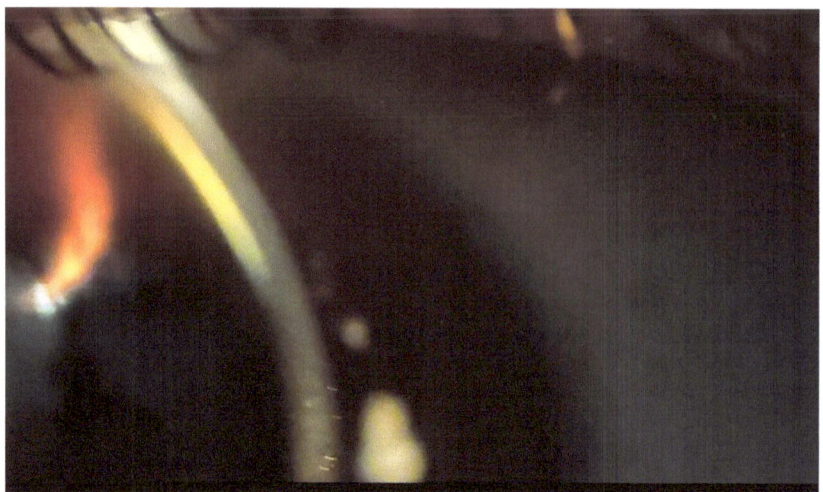

Figure 20 (b): Slit-lamp examination lateral view showing Kayser Fleischer ring in the same patient.
(Photograph by Sharjeel M)

VASCULAR PATHOLOGY

Nazli Gul

Retina has a dual blood supply which is derived from the branches of ophthalmic artery i.e. the central retinal artery and the posterior ciliary arteries.

Central retinal artery supplies the inner $2/3^{rd}$ whereas the posterior ciliary arteries supply the outer $1/3^{rd}$ of the retina and choroid.

The central retinal artery and vein with their branches are normally visible in the fundus.

Occlusion of these vessels may affect the blood supply and drainage of the retina and these changes can easily be seen on fundoscopy.

Some of the possible scenarios are given below.

RETINAL ARTERY OCCLUSION

Occlusion of the central retinal artery (CRAO) is an ocular emergency and if treated in time, it may prevent the irreversible visual loss.

The two important risk factors are atherosclerosis-related thrombosis and carotid embolism.

The risk of stroke is relatively high in the first few weeks following retinal arterial occlusion.

CRAO causes ischemia of the whole retina and the patient presents with sudden and profound painless loss of vision.

In patients with patent cilioretinal artery, the central vision may be preserved.

FUNDOSCOPIC FINDINGS

The whole retina is whitish and edematous except for the normal pink retina temporal to the optic disc and a cherry red spot at the macula due to patent cilio-retinal artery.

BPRANCH RETINAL ARTERY OCCLUSION

Occlusion of a branch of the central retinal artery (BRAO) also presents with sudden profound painless visual loss.

Arterial occlusion is visible in the fundus as whitish edematous retina. (Fig. 21, 22)

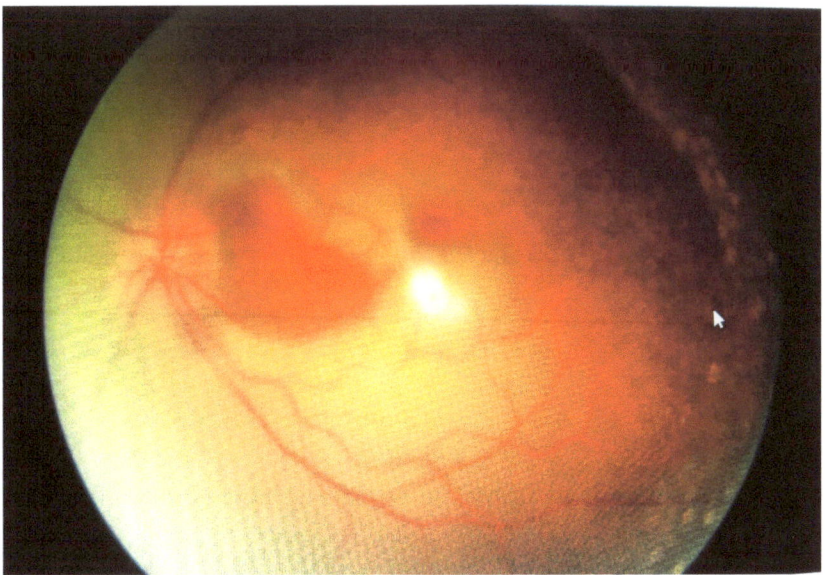

Figure 21: Central retinal artery occlusion leading to whitish edematous retina. The normal pink retina temporal to the optic disc and a cherry red spot at the macula is due to patent cilioretinal artery.
(Fundus photograph by Sharjeel M)

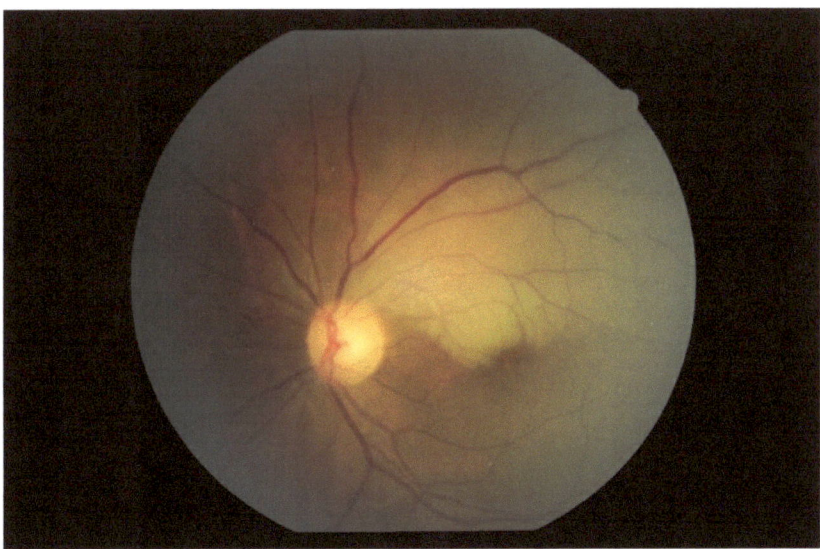

Figure 22: Branch retinal artery occlusion leading to pallor of the upper temporal quadrant of the fundus.
(Fundus photograph by Khalid K)

RETINAL VEIN OCCLUSION

Occlusion of the central retinal vein (CRVO) also leads to sudden, severe, painless, loss of vision.

It commonly occurs in those over 65 years of age but up to 15% may affect the patients under 45. Important risk factors include hypertension, dyslipidemia, diabetes, smoking, glaucoma and oral contraceptive pills.

In younger patients, thrombophilia screening and autoantibodies testing should be requested. Patients with retinal vein occlusion in one eye has an increased incidence of this occurring in the other one as well.

On fundoscopy, there is dilatation and tortuosity of all the branches of central retinal vein, extensive retinal hemorrhages, cotton wool spots and optic disc hyperemia or edema. (Fig. 23)

BRANCH RETINAL VEIN OCCLUSION

Occlusion of a branch of the central retinal vein (BRVO) may also cause sudden onset painless blurring of vision. However, the patient may be asymptomatic if peripheral branch of the vein is occluded.

On fundoscopy, there is dilatation and tortuosity of the affected vein, retinal hemorrhages and cotton wool spots in the part of retina drained by the obstructed branch of the vein. (Fig. 24)

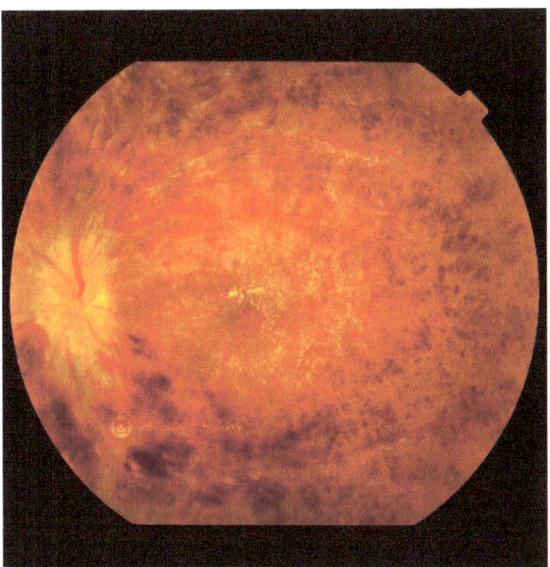

Figure 23: Central retinal vein occlusion with venous dilatation & tortuosity and retinal hemorrhages of the whole retina.
(Fundus photograph by Sharjeel M)

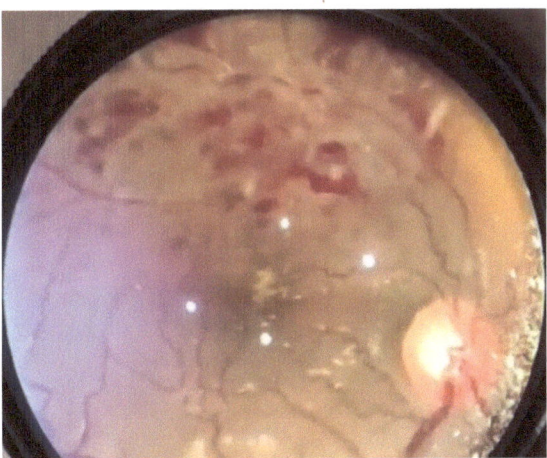

Figure 24: Branch retinal vein occlusion with venous congestion and hemorrhages in the upper temporal quadrant.
(Fundus photograph by Sharjeel M)

MILIARY TUBERCULOSIS

Khan H

Tuberculosis is quite common in the developing countries. Its usual diagnosis is based on sputum AFB &/or chest x-ray findings in case of pulmonary and tissue diagnosis for the extra-pulmonary TB. In rare circumstances tubercles can be observed on fundoscopy in patients with miliary tuberculosis.

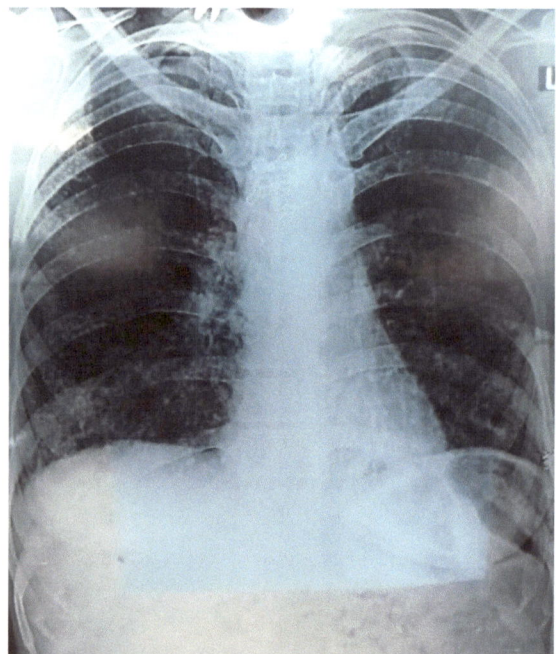

Figure 25: Chest x-ray of a patient with miliary tuberculosis showing milliary mottling throughout both the lung fields. (Photograph by Khan H)

INFECTIVE ENDOCARDITIS

Khan H

Infective endocarditis is a serious condition with significant morbidity and mortality. Prompt diagnosis and treatment are essential to minimize its sequelae.

Endocarditis is usually the consequence of two factors:

1. Abnormal endocardium
2. Bacteremia

Certain procedures lead to bacteremia, e.g. orodental, upper & lower GI, or genito-urinary procedures.

Organisms commonly involved are Streptococcus epidermidis, other Streptococcal spp. and Staphylococcus aureus.

CLINICAL FEATURES

Fever with changing murmur (±Haematuria /splenomegaly) is infective endocarditis unless proved otherwise.

Subacute bacterial endocarditis (SBE) may have the following features:

1. Infective: Fever, weight loss, malaise, night sweats, clubbing, splenomegaly and anaemia.
2. Heart murmurs due to valvular insufficiency, which may progress to intractable congestive cardiac failure and myocardial abscesses.
3. Embolic: Mycotic aneurysms and stroke.
4. Vasculitic: Microscopic haematuria, splinter haemorrhages, Osler's nodes, Janeway lesions, Roth spots, and renal impairment.

INVESTIGATIONS

Blood culture - Blood culture - Blood culture:

Three cultures at different times and from different veins, preferably when fever is rising.

Echocardiography:

Transthorasic echo may show vegetations >3 mm. Transesophageal echocardiography (TOE) is more sensitive.

Fundoscopy:

Typical Roth spots may be seen. (Fig. 26) Roth spots are actually hemorrhagic spots with central clearing.

Streptococcus bovis endocarditis may be associated with colonic carcinoma and should prompt colonoscopy.

MANAGEMENT

Parenteral antibiotics like Penicillin G + Streptomycin or Gentamycin for 2 weeks. Ceftriaxone or Vancomycin for penicillin resistant streptococci for 4 weeks.

Consider surgery e.g. valve replacement (under Strep cover) if worsening LVF.

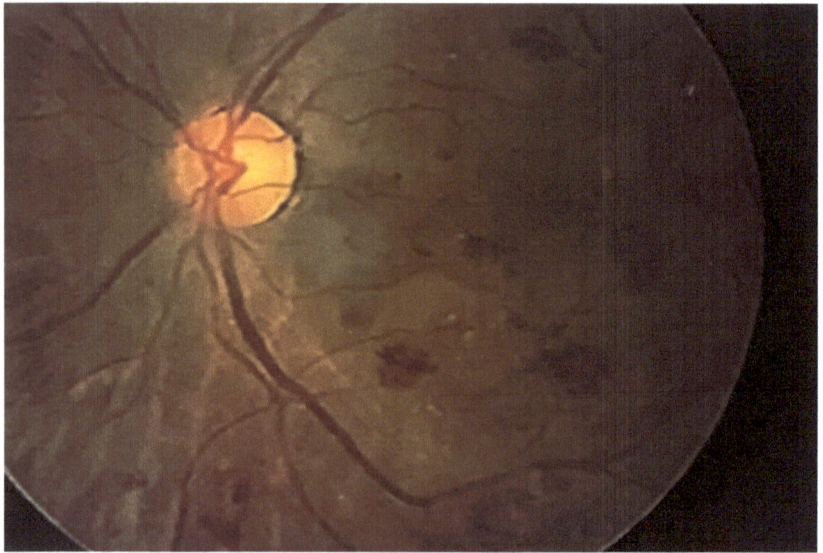

Figure 26: Fundus showing multiple Roth spots in a 55 years old Afghan lady with CML having septicemia.
(Fundus photograph by Ilyas MA & Sharjeel M)

PROPHYLAXIS

Indications:
1. Previous history of infective endocarditis
2. Rheumatic heart disease.
3. Congenital: Most forms with exception like MVP without MR.
4. Degenerative heart disease.
5. Prosthetic valves and other intravascular prostheses.
6. Hypertrophic cardiomyopathy.

Procedures requiring Endocarditis prophylaxis:
All procedures leading to significant bacteremia.

PROGNOSIS
If left untreated, infective endocarditis is almost inevitably fatal.

HEMATOLOGICAL DISORDERS

Habib H

Various hematological disorders can affect the fundus and show characteristic changes.

Some examples are given below.

ANEMIA

Deficiency of hemoglobin or RBCs. It can be classified on the basis of morphology into Microcytic, Macrocytic, or Normocytic.

Microcytic anemia is commonly due to iron deficiency, thallassemia, or sideroblastic.

Macrocytic anemia is due to vitamin B12 or folate deficiency.

Normocytic anemia is due to chronic disease like chronic renal failure.

The optic disc is obviously pale in severe anemia. Other changes depend upon the cause of anemia. (Fig. 27)

LEUKEMIA

Leukemia is the neoplastic condition of WBCs or precursor cells. It can be acute or chronic.

The fundi may show hemorrhages because of the thrombocytopenia usually present in these patients. (Fig. 27)

Leukemic deposits may also be sometimes visible in the fundus. In patients with septicemia the typical Roth spots as in infective endocarditis may be visible.

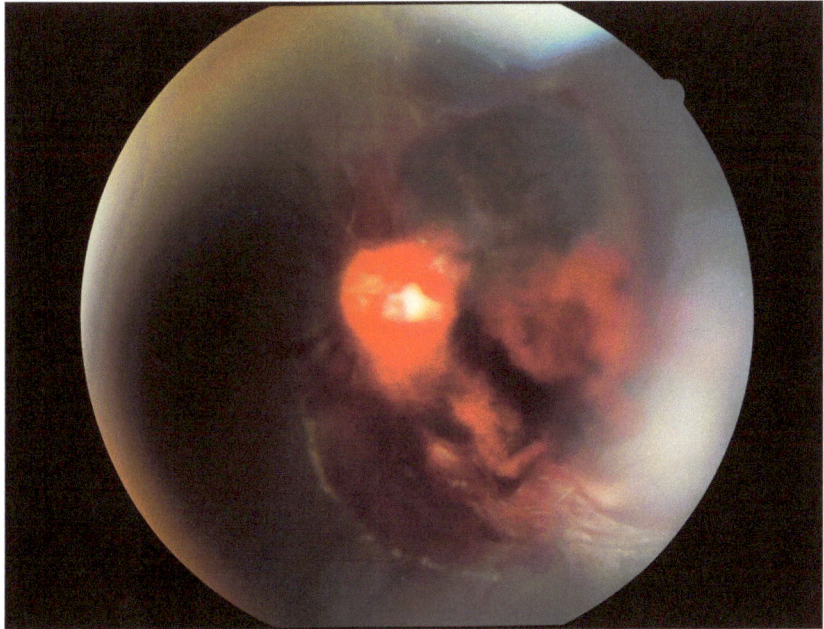

Figure 27: Pre-retinal hemorrhage in a patient with thalassemia.
(Fundus photograph by Khalid K)

SYSTEMIC LUPUS ERYTHEMATOSUS

Habib H

Systemic lupus erythematosus (SLE) is an autoimmune disorder which can affect any organ system of the body including the eyes. Lupus nephritis is the most serious manifestation of SLE.

The diagnosis of SLE is based on at least 4 out of 11 criteria of the American College of Rheumatology (ACR). (Table 4)

Retinal involvement is the most common ocular manifestation and lupus retinopathy should alert the clinicians to the likelihood of systemic vasculitic lesions requiring aggressive systemic therapy.

There may be macular edema and intraretinal hemorrhages and cotton-wool spots indistinguishable from hypertensive retinopathy and it may be impossible to decide whether these lesions are just due to hypertension or SLE immune complex vasculitis.

Aggressive therapy for HT and SLE is associated with dramatic decrease in these retinal lesions. Episcleritis and scleritis may occur in SLE and it is also a reasonably accurate guide to the presence of significant systemic activity. It resolves with control of disease activity.

SLE can also cause keratitis, and choroidopathy which may lead to retinal detachment.

As SLE patients are on long-term HCQ, one must be vigilant to detect its toxic effects as early as possible. These include irreversible retinopathy with pigmentation changes at the macula (Bull's eye appearance).

ACR DIAGNOSTIC CRITERIA FOR SLE

SOAP	BRAIN	MD
1. **S**erositis 2. **O**ral ulcers 3. **A**rthritis 4. **P**hotosensitivity	5. **B**lood disorders 6. **R**enal involvement 7. **A**NA 8. **I**mmunologic phenomena 9. **N**eurologic disorder	10. **M**alar rash 11. **D**iscoid rash

Table 4: Mnemonic for the ACR diagnostic criteria of SLE.
Key: ACR - American College of Rheumatology, ANA - Anti-nuclear antibodies, SLE - Systemic lupus erythematosus.

CONNECTIVE TISSUE DISORDERS

Habib H

Connective tissue disorders are a group of genetic disorders with defective formation of connective tissues which may lead to changes in the musculoskeletal and vascular system, Ii may also affect the ocular system.

Examples of such defects are:

- Pseudoxanthoma elasticum
- Ehlers Danlos syndrome
- Marfan syndrome

Ophthalmic changes in these disorders can rarely be available to be shown in the exam but a postgraduate student or a clinician must know about these changes.

PSEUDOXANTHOMA ELASTICUM

Pseudoxanthoma elasticum is a rare genetic disorder characterized by progressive calcification and fragmentation of elastic fibers affecting the skin, retina, and the cardiovascular system. Cutaneous lesions typically begin in the childhood or early adolescence, but owing to their asymptomatic nature and appearance like xanthomas, these are usually ignored. (Fig. 28)

Fundus examination may reveal angioid streaks. (Fig. 29)

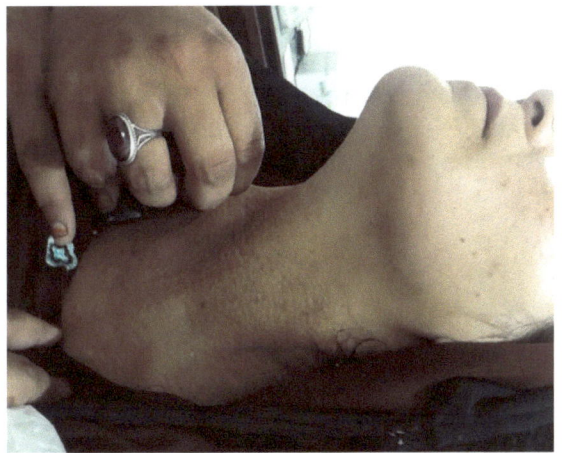

Figure 28: young lady with pseudoxanthoma elasticum; demonstrating the loose chicken-like skin.
(Photograph by Khalid K)

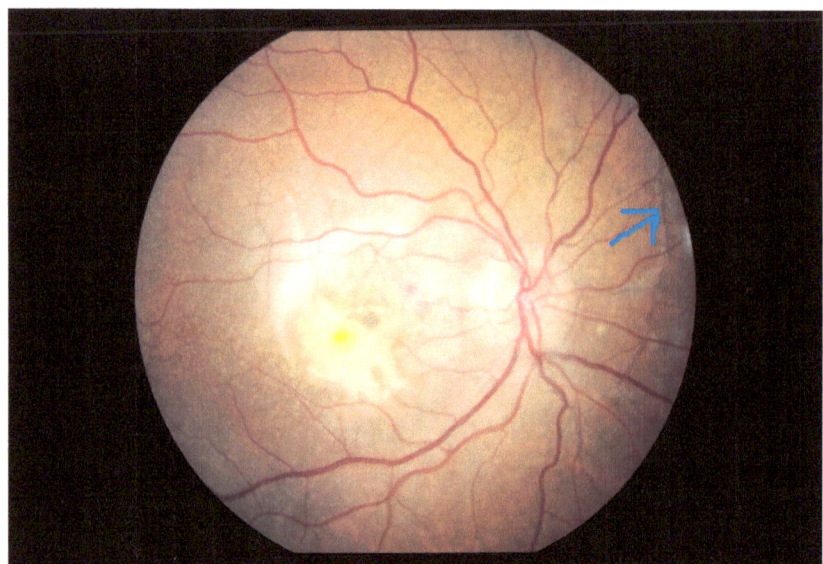

Figure 29: Fundus photo showing angioid streaks in the same patient with pseudoxanthoma elasticum. Arrow is pointing to one such streak. There is a macular scar due to choroidal neovascularization.

(Fundus photograph by Khalid K)

EHLERS DANLOS SYNDROME

Ehlers Danlos syndrome is a clinically and genetically heterogeneous group of connective-tissue disorder, involving a defect in the collagen and connective-tissue synthesis and structure. It can affect the skin, joints, and blood vessels.

Clinically it has six distinct types:

- Classical
- Vascular
- Kyphoscoliotic
- Arthrochalasis
- Dermatospraxis

Recognition of various types is important as the vascular type is associated with life-threatening arterial rupture and visceral perforation.

The eyes may show progressive thinning of the cornea (blue sclerae) and early-onset keratoglobus or keratoconus.

MARFAN SYNDROME

Marfan syndrome is an autosomal dominant hereditary disorder of connective tissues in which the skeleton shows multiple deformities like arachnodactyly i.e. abnormally long and thin digits, long limbs relative to the trunk, chest deformities (pectus excavatum or carinatum) and scoliosis.

Chest and spine abnormalities may cause restrictive lung disease and ultimate corpulmonale if left untreated.

Aortic root dilatation, aortic regurgitation, and mitral valve prolapse (MVP) can occur. Aortic root changes may lead to dissection of aorta which may be fatal.

Ocular findings include myopia, cataracts, retinal detachment, and superior dislocation of the lens with resultant glaucoma.

These ocular changes may lead to blindness if unrecognized and left untreated.

BIBLIOGRAPHY

1. Chatziralli IP, et al. The value of fundoscopy in general practice. Open Ophthalmol. J 2012; 6:4–5.
2. Gilkes MJ. The GP and the specialist ophthalmology. Br Med J. 1982; 285:1247–8.
3. Gurland BB. The GP and the ophthalmoscope. J Med Soc N J. 1964; 61:447–8.
4. Ganguly AK. Scope of ophthalmoscopy in general practice and its significance. Indian Med J. 1964; 61:39–41.
5. Turner HE, et al. Oxford Handbook of Endocrinology and Diabetes. Oxford University Press. Chapter 106.
6. James PA, et al. Evidence-based guideline for the management of high blood pressure in adults (JNC8). JAMA 2014; 311:507-20.
7. Diabetic Eye Disease. p. 286.
8. Papadakis MA, et al. Current Medical Diagnosis and Treatment. 2015. Lange McGraw Hill Education.
9. Keith N, et al. Some different types of essential hypertension: their course and prognosis. Am J Med Sci. 1939; 196:332–9.
10. Henderson AD, et al. Hypertension-related eye abnormalities and the risk of stroke. Rev Neurol Dis. 2011; 8:1–9.
11. Henderson AD, et al. Grade III or Grade IV Hypertensive retinopathy with severely elevated blood pressure. West J Emerg Med. 2012; 13:529–34.
12. Medscape. e-medicine.
13. Mayo Clinic. Diabetic retinopathy. http://www.mayoclinic.org/diseases-conditions/diabetic-retinopathy/expert-answers/con-20023311
14. Kierstan Boyd. Who Is at Risk for Diabetic Retinopathy? American Academy of Ophthalmology. Eye Health A to Z. https://www.aao.org/eye-health/diseases/diabetic-retinopathy-risk
15. Foster CS. Ocular manifestations of systemic lupus erythematosus.
16. John FS. (2020). Kanski's Clinical Ophthalmology. A Systematic Approach. 9th Edn. Elsevier Limited.
17. Zhou Y, et al. Relationship between retinal vascular occlusions and incident cerebrovascular diseases: a systematic review and meta-analysis. Medicine (Baltimore). 2016 Jun; 95(26): e4075.
18. Central Vein Occlusion Study Group. Baseline and early natural history report: the Central Vein Occlusion Study. Arch Ophthalmol. 1993; 111:1087-95.
19. Rogers S, et al. International Eye Disease Consortium. The prevalence of retinal vein

occlusion: pooled data from population studies from the United States, Europe, Asia, and Australia. Ophthalmology. 2010; 117:313-9.

20. Central Vein Occlusion Study Group. Natural history and clinical management of central retinal vein occlusion. Arch Ophthalmol. 1997; 115:486-91.

21. Hayreh SS, et al. Incidence of various types of retinal vein occlusion and their recurrence and demographic characteristics. Am J Ophthalmol. 1994; 117:429-41.

22. Armstrong C. JNC 8 Guidelines for the management of hypertension in adults. Am Fam Physician. 2014; 90:503-4.

ABOUT THE AUTHOR

Habibullah Khan

Professor Habibullah Khan, a graduate of Khyber Medical College, Peshawar; Member of the College of Physicians & Surgeons of Pakistan, and Fellow of the Royal College of Physicians of Edinburgh, UK; is presently working as Consultant Physician at Rauf Medical Centre, D.I.Khan, Pakistan.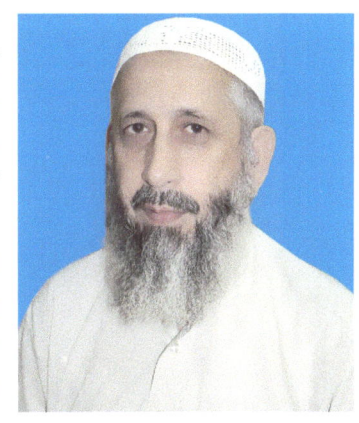
He worked as Professor of Medicine at Gomal Medical College, D.I.Khan. He has also served at various health sectors in the country and abroad including Army Medical Corps, Provincial Health Services, Kingdom of Saudi Arabia, and United Kingdom.

He is enthusiastically involved in research and has published more than 70 papers. He has also authored a book "PEARLS OF MEDICINE - LONG CASE" available at Amazon.

During his services at GMC he initiated the research journal, "Gomal Journal of Medical Sciences" which is one of the internationally recognized and renounced medical serial.

BOOKS BY THIS AUTHOR

Pearls Of Medicine: Long Case

This book is basically an aid to prepare for the long-case in the clinical examinations of Internal Medicine & allied subjects. Long-case is an integral component of any clinical examination and its purpose is to check whether the candidate is prepared enough to deal with the patients in a safe and logical way. This work will help not only the students to go through their clinical exams successfully but will also be an aid for the practicing physicians.

www.ingramcontent.com/pod-product-compliance
Lightning Source LLC
Chambersburg PA
CBHW051159220526
45473CB00003B/834